MW00336024

PROSPER AND BE IN HEALTH...

GEMS FOR WELLNESS ATTRACTION

by Dr. Gayle Jones, N.D., R.N.

Published by Wellness Attraction Enterprises LLC

Prosper and Be in Health...Gems for Wellness Attraction

by Dr. Gayle Jones, N.D., R.N.

Published by Wellness Attraction Enterprises LLC

3540 Crain Highway #415

Bowie, Maryland 20716

www.WellnessAttraction.com

First Printing, 2015

ISBN: 978-0692508589

Neither the publisher nor the author is engaged in rendering professional advice or services to the reader. The principles, ideas and suggestions in this book are not intended as a substitute for consulting with your health care provider. Neither the author nor the publisher shall be liable or responsible for any loss or damage allegedly arising from any information or suggestion in the book.

Table of Contents

ACKNOWLEDGMENTS

To God be the glory for the GREAT things He has done! Thank You God, for giving me the tongue of the learned that I should know how to speak a Word in Season to those who are weary (Isaiah 50:4)

Loving gratitude to my treasured husband for supporting and loving me in innumerable ways so that I could complete this important assignment;

Thank You Lord for giving us loving jewels in the persons of our cherished daughters Nicole and Brittany and our precious grandson, Landon. You are loved and treasured so much! Special thanks to Brittany for her technologic skills that produced this book by the publishing deadline.

Thank You Heavenly Father for giving me the BEST earthly father, who is now in Your presence (Dr. Samuel L. Banks), who lovingly referred to me and my sister as his JEWELS and treasured us as such.

Many thanks to my wonderful mother (Elizabeth Banks) for laying a foundation of love, wisdom and wellness attraction in my life.

Special thanks to my dear sister/best friend, Allison for keeping me on point and yet encouraging me to complete this God-inspired literary work; Gratitude to my "Sweet, Smart Niece" Faith for all of her special comments that confirmed my divine assignment to write this book;

Special thanks to my "Earth Angel" Minister Patricia Grantham for always being obedient to God's call to love and help me, always right on time, from childhood through adulthood! Thank you for all of your support in the publishing of this God-inspired literary work.

Special thanks to Donna Rivers for years of effectual prayers for me and speaking into existence amazing possibilities for my life.

Eternal gratitude to my quintessential Pastor John K, Jenkins, Sr. and First Lady Trina Jenkins for being anointed servant leaders after God's own heart. Your Biblically-based instruction, humility and servant leadership continue to inspire me to be a dynamic disciple locally, nationally and internationally.

Special thanks to Rev. Esther Gordon for giving me the privilege of utilizing my gifts to teach Nutrition and Healthy Living in The Institutes at the First Baptist Church of Glenarden. This book is documented fruit from that class.

Special thanks to Mary Brown for faithfully inspiring me to share God's Word with those who need medicine that heals the spirit, soul and body.

Thanks to Dr. Fred Jones, Esq. for the effective, inaugural *Publish Me Now Retreat* that laid a great foundation for me becoming an impactful author.

Special thanks to my brilliant G.E.M.S. (Gayle's Excellent Mentors): Rev. Belynda Gentry, Debra Townsend-York, Marshawn Evans Daniels and Jack Daniels for being inspirational and shining brightly in my life as my faith/business mentors!

Special thanks to my G.E.M.S (Gayle's Excellent Mentees): Jade Slaffey, Kendra Brown, Allison Tucker, and Ethel Kemp Wade, who challenge me to continue to grow as a life-long learner.

I acknowledge you, the reader and say "thank you" for investing in this book and being a doer of the Word. God created you to be a G.E.M….God's Excellent Model of prosperity and health in your spirit, soul and body, throughout your lifetime. Shine forth!

Introduction

I will praise thee for I am fearfully and wonderfully made; Marvelous are your works, and that my soul knows very well. (Psalm 139:14)

There is an abundance of information available concerning health and wellness. It can therefore, be a daunting task to try to discover the correct path of wellness for oneself. With the increasing incidences of health problems such as Type-2 Diabetes, Cardiovascular Disease and certain cancers, it is imperative to create the environment for wellness attraction ideally before sickness and disease manifest. If disease has already manifested, the steps for creating an environment for wellness attraction should begin immediately.

College students can benefit from creating the environment for wellness attraction before entering campus life and while being a college student. Young marrieds can benefit from creating an environment of wellness attraction before becoming parents. A newly pregnant woman can benefit from creating an environment of wellness attraction in order to be a healthy "incubator" for the baby developing inside of her. Parents can benefit from creating an environment of wellness attraction so that they can live well and nurture children not besieged by generational health curses and societal pollution. The young adult can benefit from creating the environment for wellness attraction as he or she lives healthy through their years and stages of maturity even into the stage of menopause, andropause and beyond! Employers surely can benefit from exposing their employees and their families to winning wellness attraction principles, which lead to a healthier, happier and more productive work force and less absences and family leave due to illness. There are many accounts of centenarians who have followed health wisdom and continue to attract wellness into their lives.

As a registered nurse working in an environment where children/teens came for emergencies and urgent care problems, I was regularly in the midst of crises and illness. However, in 35 years of being in that environment, I maintained an impeccable work attendance record, because I remained well! I did not take the flu shot and never contracted the flu, even while caring for thousands of sick children/teens. At 58 years of age, my primary care physician marvels at the fact that I am not on any medications. I value the gift of health that God has given me as well as the health wisdom that HE has imparted to me throughout my life.

God desires that we be in health. At the point of creation, God breathed into man the breath of life and man became a living soul. Our fearfully and wonderfully made bodies were created for optimal functioning to carry out our unique God-given purposes. I am pleased to share with you how you can translate health knowledge into health wisdom for your fearfully and wonderfully made body. Get ready to excavate the gems for attracting

wellness to your life and creating your unique care plan to….
Prosper and Be in Health!

Spirit Wellness

And you shall love the Lord your God out of and with your whole heart and out of and with all your soul (your life) and out of and with all of your mind (with your faculty of thought and your moral understanding) and out of and with all of your strength all will all of your soul and with all of your strength. This is the first and principle commandment. This is the first and principal commandment.

Mark 12:30 (AMP)

Love GOD

The truth is that each person is first spirit, has a soul (which comprises the mind, will and emotions) and lives in a body. God created the body in such an amazing way. It is important to remain in contact with the One who created us and who loves His creation! In remaining in contact with God, we can have spirit wellness! Spirit wellness requires an understanding that it is in God that we live, move and have our being!

Prayer time

I am happily married, am a mother, and grandmother. However, my first spoken words, before I speak to anyone else, are to God as a whisper prayer. I pray, the moment I open my eyes each day. Prayer is my vital two-way communication with God. I do have a planner that details my tentative daily agenda. However, I have learned in my "Quiet Time" with Him each day. As I talk to God and listen to Him, He confirms and orders my steps!

Throughout my day, I pray. As I drove to work, I definitely had to remain prayerful…."Lord, help me not to be affected by these drivers with road rage."

"Lord, help me to remain calm and not call the driver who just cut me off in traffic an unkind name!" (I used to say, "Knuckle head!")

As a former pediatric emergency/trauma nurse, I prayed silently to myself while an upset parent stood in front of me yelling because their child with a rash wasn't getting medical attention fast enough in the emergency room. I can recall one occasion in which I prayed asking God to give me the correct words in Spanish to say to a frightened family in the intensive care unit whose child was dying. Over the course of my nursing career, I have prayed for wisdom for the physicians and my other colleagues, so that we could implement the appropriate care for every ill or injured child in our circles of influence.

Benefits of Prayer

❖ Prayer enhances one's intimate relationship with God.
❖ Prayer provides Divine wisdom. God is omniscient, however, God delights in hearing one's requests for deliverance and guidance. (Jeremiah 33:3)
❖ Prayer enables one to be less "ME-focused" and more "others focused" as one focuses on the needs of others. (James 5:16)
❖ Those who are emotionally and physically healthy have prayer as an important part of their healthy lifestyle.

Worship has been linked to lowering blood pressure and strengthening the immune system.

❖ Praying regularly reduces stress as one casts all of one's cares on the Lord. (1 Peter 5:7)

❖ Praying is communication with God in which we can confess our sins and gain forgiveness. 1 John 1:9 states that "If we confess our sins, He is faithful and just to forgive us our sins, and to cleanse us from all unrighteousness.

❖ Prayer improves one's attitudes. Humility enters in as one realizes one's need for God. (Matthew 24:42)

❖ Prayer can keep one from entering into temptation. (Matthew 24:42)

❖ Prayer strengthens one as God gives direction, answers prayer and gives one the ability to stand strong during difficult times.

❖ Prayer builds one up spiritually. (Jude 1:20)

Prayer is one of the gems for wellness attraction that enables one to receive specific health wisdom.

GEMS for Spirit Wellness

❖ Begin your day with communication with God (prayer). Thank God for your relationship with Him. Thank God that you have a mind to acknowledge and serve Him. Thank God for your fearfully and wonderfully made body....your abilities (to breathe, to live). Spend more time seeking and listening to God. As you read the Bible, allow scriptures to become alive in you.

❖ Ask God to reveal your unique care plan for prospering and being in health.

❖ Bible study and memorization is foundational to spiritual wellness. We function optimally when we have a well-toned spirit man in a fit and well-toned body. Remember the truth that we are spirit, we have a soul (mind, will and emotions) and we live in a body.

One way to think about this is utilizing the analogy of a car and gasoline. In the car owner's manual, are found the manufacturer's specifications for what type of gas and preventive maintenance will give optimal performance for a car. It is a fact that most expensive, high performance cars use high octane gas and go through costly maintenance.

Similarly, God originally placed high octane fuel in the form of good nutritional food for us, both spiritually and physically. If we fail to fuel our spirit and soul (mind, will and emotions) with the best fuel (staying full and not on empty!), we will not function at an optimal level of wellness. If we continue to drive our bodies on less than optimal fuel, eventually the body breaks down just as a car will! God's Word is the Manual for living well. It contains the jewels of wisdom for optimal spirit wellness!

Praise and Worship

Psalm 150:6 states, "Let everything that has breath, praise the Lord"! All of creation abounds with praise to God, the Sovereign Creator! Early in the morning, the birds are melodiously singing with their chirps of praise to the One who made them. The seas roar with the power and majesty of magnificent waves of water.

God breathed into man His breath of life. Therefore, as Psalm 150 states let every living thing that has breath, praise the Lord! Praise God by talking about His goodness. Worship God by proclaiming how awesome He really is in our lives. Worship Him in obedience to His word. Worship Him by having a lifestyle of prayer. Worship Him in a place of solitude and worship Him corporately with other true worshippers. Regular praise and worship is a gem for wellness attraction for optimal spirit wellness.

I wake up every morning with praise and worship to God. I have a lifestyle of praise. I praise and worship him in my home. One of my favorite places for praise and worship is outside near the water on a warm sunny day. I experience creation praising God with the swell of the waves of the sea, the sea gulls bird calls, and the warm breezes blowing occasionally on my skin.

Our first born daughter, as an infant would get up like clockwork at 3:00 am every morning. She would cry and cry. Even after having her hunger satisfied, she refused to go back to sleep! She didn't care that I was ready to go back to sleep! Therefore, her nursery would transform into a sanctuary of praise and worship as I rocked her in my arms and thanked God that she was a healthy infant. In the wee hours of the morning I thanked God for the high calling of motherhood! Yes, I rocked her in our rocking chair while God rocked me as I talked and sang worship songs to Him.

Praise and worship is best as a lifestyle. When I worked as an emergency/trauma nurse for children, those were busy days in the hospital. However, when I had an opportunity for a break, I would go to my car, which was parked in the parking garage on the lower level of the hospital. There I would turn on praise music in my car, pray and be renewed in the presence of God. My car became a sanctuary and a vehicle of restoration for me.

God is present everywhere. He can be praised and worshipped by a young mother or father cradling their infant and singing. He can be praised by employees during a lunch break at work. God can be praised near the waters of a beach or inside the walls of a church building. Yes, being in relationship with God and implementing the disciplines for being healthy in one's spirit are essential wellness attraction gems.

If all of the previous information sounds foreign to you and you'd like to be an eternal part of Gods' family, I'd like to introduce you to the One who can enable you to prosper and be in health even as your soul (mind, will and emotions) prosper (3 John 2). Wellness in one's spirit, is foundational for the soul and body to prosper and be in health. I invite you with all sincerity, to recite aloud the following prayer:

Dear God, I know that I am a sinner. I need a Savior who I believe is Your Son Jesus. Jesus is the only way that I can have a relationship with You forever. I want to be a part of Your family. I want to prosper and be in health in my spirit, soul and body so that I can have Your power to carry out the wonderful plans that you have for my life. Thank you Jesus for dying on the cross for my sins. Not only did You die for me, but I believe that God raised you from the dead. I want that same awesome power to be in me. Thank You for hearing, saving and loving me! Thank You God that I am Your Daughter/Son! Thank You Holy Spirit that You have come to live in me! Thank You Jesus that You are now Lord of my life!

Tools for Excavating GEMS of Wellness for your spirit: Bible, notebook for recording notes from sermons, biblical lessons, membership in Bible-teaching church

Here are some study nuggets. As you read/meditate on verses from the Bible, ask yourself the following questions:

- ❖ What attribute(s) (qualities, characteristics) of God are displayed?
- ❖ What gems of truth are being revealed?
- ❖ Is there a behavior of the biblical characters that I need to or need not to imitate?
- ❖ What unique message am I hearing from reading/meditating on this verse(s)?

Soul (Mind, Will & Emotions) Wellness

The Bible states "As a man thinks so is he". Therefore, it is important that we have "soul wellness". The soul is that part of us that includes the mind, will and emotions.

Have you ever been around anyone who hears the public announcement that it is Flu Season and immediately they start saying negative things? For example they may say, "It's Flu Season and I know I'm going to get it because I always get sick." Another example is how some people embrace and are possessive of an illness by innocently saying, "**My** asthma is acting up right now." or "**My** pre-diabetes will probably turn into full-blown diabetes because my grandmother died from it and my mother has it." An important Biblically-based GEM for soul wellness is, "...For out of the abundance (overflow) of the heart his mouth speaks." (Luke 6:45). Be watchful and very selective concerning what enters the eye gates, the ear gates, the heart gates and the mind gates.

out of the good treasure of his heart brings forth good...

An important Bible Gem for soul wellness is, "Out of the abundance of the heart the mouth speaks." (Matt 12:34) Therefore, it is critical that one be watchful and very selective concerning what enters the eye gate, the ear gate, the heart gate and the mind gate, and be even more selective of what comes out of the mouth gate. I will elaborate on the following 3 areas concerning soul wellness:

- ❖ Controlling Your Thought Life, What comes in your "Gates" (what you see, what you hear)
- ❖ Forgiveness (Self & Others)
- ❖ Stress Management

Controlling Your Thought Life

Do not be conformed to this world (this age), [fashioned after and adapting to its external, superficial customs], but be transformed (changed) by the [entire] renewal of your mind [by its new ideals and its new attitude] so that you may prove [for yourselves] what is the good and acceptable and perfect will of God, even the thing which is good and acceptable and perfect [in His sight for you]

Romans 12:2 (AMP)

What we think about inwardly gets manifested outwardly. Therefore, if negative or erroneous information has been living in our minds without paying any rent, it's time to evict those negative thoughts! Whenever a negative or erroneous thought comes to our mind's front door, immediately discard the thought and replace it with what God says about the situation. Renewing our mind doesn't mean getting a completely new brain so to speak. It means lining our thoughts back up with God's original ways, thoughts, purposes and plans for us.

When my father had 3 heart attacks, and his pessimistic cardiologist told us that my father needed a heart transplant and even with that would only likely live for a year, we had to immediately start renewing our minds with God's word on healing. Day and night my mother, sister and I listened to faith-based cassettes. We played them for ourselves and in the hospital room where my Dad was. It was already our lifestyle to "pray without ceasing", and we continued to do so. We heard the report of the cardiologist, but the voice of God's Word was louder!

My father had a third heart attack while still in the hospital. Yet we remained steadfast in renewing our minds with the Word of God, and we watched our confessions. A competent and confident Jewish cardio-thoracic surgeon spoke up and said "I believe that I can do by-pass surgery on this man." The triple by-pass surgery was successful! God added 7 years (God's perfect number) to the 1 year that the pessimistic cardiologist gave in his limited report. Seven plus one is eight which is the number of new beginning! God's grace and the power of His Word was and still is …more than enough!

We must always guard our thoughts and what comes into our minds, our ears and what comes in and out of our mouths! The Bible says that out of the abundance of our hearts the mouth speaks!

GEMS for Soul Wellness

Guard what enters the gates of your eyes, ears, heart and mouth

❖ Control what enters the "gates" of your eyes, ears, heart and mouth. Get rid of mindless television viewing. Be intentional about allowing only good/wholesome information to come into your eyes, mouth and ears. Fill your mind with the word of God, wisdom, positive thoughts and beneficial information/education. Refuse to let negative emotions like bitterness, revenge, resentment, rage, envy, and evil fill your mind and heart.

❖ Let your renewed mind be a filter that closely examines the kinds of information that you see or hear. If it's negative, corrupt or unhealthy in any way turn it off and move away from it. If you can't move away, tune it out and close your ears and heart to it.

❖ Be selective about the type of music that is around you. Classical music is calming to the spirit of a crying infant and brings peace to an environment. A room blaring with television noises, loud radio, and loud voices can be irritating to one's spirit.

❖ Let no corrupt communication come forth from your mouth. Avoid listening to gossip and spreading gossip.

❖ Clear clutter from your living environment. When your eyes see a non-cluttered, beautiful environment it sets the stage for creativity, excellence and wellness to come forth in your speech and your work. Sleep is better in a non-cluttered, peaceful bedroom.

❖ Take time to visit places of beauty such as an art museum/art gallery, beautiful natural outdoor settings during the different seasons and visit botanical gardens. Gaze at beautiful books of art.

❖ Pray the Scriptures aloud. Personalize the Scriptures. (Example of a personalized prayer using Psalm 23: "Thank You Lord that You are my Shepherd and I shall not want. You allow me to lie down in green pastures. Thank You for restoring my soul. Thank You for leading me in the paths of righteousness for Your names' sake.)

Tools for Excavating GEMS of Wellness for your Soul (mind, will and emotions):

The Bible, inspirational books/readings, active membership in a faith community, loving family and supportive relationships, inspirational music, beautiful surroundings in nature/home/art museum

Forgiveness

I thank God that while I was still yet a sinner, Christ died for me (Romans 5:8)! I am thankful that when I disobey God and confess my sin to Him, He is faithful and just to forgive me and cleanse me from all unrighteousness. So freely I have been forgiven and so freely I must forgive others!

In the course of life, we will have experiences where people betray and hurt us in unintentional and intentional ways. I have learned that forgiveness is required whether the person who has hurt me asks for forgiveness or not! I have learned that there is freedom in forgiving my seen and unseen enemies!

The condition of our heart regarding forgiving others affects our mental and physical health. Harboring unforgiveness in one's heart has been linked to stress-related disorders and some cancers. Daily, I review my day for any situations in which I may need to extend forgiveness. I sleep well when there is no unforgiveness in my heart. I don't want to have to be concerned about avoiding someone because someone has betrayed or hurt me.

GEMS for Soul Wellness (Forgiveness)

- ❖ Daily confess sins to God in prayer. Know that God forgives!
- ❖ If wronged by someone, seek to resolve the situation, as SOON as possible!
- ❖ Remember the adage that says that unforgiveness is like drinking poison yourself while expecting the person who wronged you to die. Don't allow unforgiveness to grow into bitterness in your heart!

Stress Management

As a registered nurse in an often high-census level three pediatric emergency medical trauma center, I adjusted to the ebb and flow of stress. Many people often asked me how I worked for twenty years caring for ill or injured children and their families in that type of environment. My answer, I know that I was called to do that very special work that I enjoyed so much!

I began working eight-hour night shifts as a new graduate nurse in that Emergency Medical Trauma Center (E.M.T.C). I remember responding to the urgent voice of the paramedic in the Emergency Command Information Center sometimes multiple times in a shift. With agility and skill, we would run next door and approach a huge helicopter where a critically ill or injured child awaited to be transported to the E.M.T.C. I vividly remember the demands on me to be a productive member of the team attempting to restore a heartbeat and the breath of life into the lifeless body of a child who had drowned. In the EMTC there were great demands on me to be a productive member of the team and many stressful encounters. There were times that a normally 30-minute lunch or dinner break would be shortened to 5 minutes. Emergencies didn't wait until I had finished eating or had finished praying in the hospital chapel, during a break. It was so important for me to take times to refresh myself and get breaks away from the demands of working as an emergency/trauma nurse.

I generally ate healthy food that had been prepared at home. I never left home without eating a healthy breakfast. Even while working 8-hour night shifts as a single, 23-year old, I could easily drive home and go directly to sleep for 8 solid hours. The hospital chapel would be the place I would go during a short break to pray and read the Bible for restoration. Lunch time was a time to eat alone or with my colleagues. However, if no one could join me for lunch, I would go to my car which was parked in the hospital garage. I turned on praise/worship music and made my car a sanctuary of relaxation, praise and restoration!

GEMS for Stress Management

❖ Recognize your stress signals that you are in "constant stress mode". Some of those signals could be "emotional eating" (eating so called "comfort foods" in order to "feel better"), being easily provoked to fits of yelling, feeling tension and pains in the neck, shoulder etc., and feeling jittery accompanied by habits like nail-biting, rapid breathing etc.

❖ Set aside time every day to relax and be rejuvenated. Make a list of activities that you enjoy that cause you to unwind and feel refreshed. Some of those activities could include: praying (Cast your cares on the Lord as it states in 1 Peter 5:7.), aerobic exercises like brisk walking or jogging, dancing for 30 minutes or more to upbeat music, drinking a warm cup of Chamomile tea, reading/meditating on inspirational verses/prose, doing something fun with someone you love, getting a massage with pure essential oils, using a diffuser of pure essential oils to infuse the air with healing aromas;

❖ Practice deep-breathing (particularly when feeling stressed) by breathing in through your nose (causing the stomach to expand) and slowly exhaling through your mouth.

❖ Have a regular bed-time routine and get ample sleep every night (or every day for those who work the night shift).

❖ Declutter your physical environment (home, office, car, dorm room). Declutter your mind of toxic, stressful thoughts. Declutter your life of negative people and negative influences.

Tools for Excavating GEMS of Wellness for your Soul (Stress Management):

The Bible, inspirational books/readings, being active in a faith community, massages, aroma therapy, aerobic exercise, peaceful music/sounds of nature, prayer

Body Wellness

So much emphasis is placed on physical body wellness. However, it is important to realize that we are tri-partite beings. We are SPIRIT, we have a SOUL (mind, will and emotions) and we live in a BODY. Thus far, we have looked at spirit wellness and soul wellness. I will address the following 5 areas that are fundamental in maintaining Body wellness:

- ❖ Nutrition
- ❖ Detoxification (fasting, proper elimination, avoiding toxins)
- ❖ Hydration
- ❖ Rest
- ❖ Movement

Nutrition

God created the world for man. He created everything for man to be well in his spirit, soul and body. God created our bodies fearfully and wonderfully and blew His breath of life into us. He lives in us because our bodies are the temple of the Holy Spirit.

"Do you not know that your body is the temple (the very sanctuary) of the Holy Spirit Who lives within you, Whom you have received (as a Gift) from God? You are not your own.

You were bought with a price purchased with a preciousness and paid for, made His own). So then, honor God and bring glory to Him in your body.

1 Corinthians 6:19, 20 (AMP)

We do well when we fuel well. Nourishing, whole food is excellent fuel for our bodies as it creates an environment for wellness attraction. Consider the fact that many of the diseases such as cardiovascular disease, obesity, Type 2 Diabetes and some cancers are linked to poor nutrition. It is therefore, imperative to learn and pray about your best nutrition and healthy living plan.

Growing up, my mother always prepared meals for me, my younger sister (Mrs. Allison Holmes) and my late father (Dr. Samuel L. Banks). She worked full-time as an educator, but always prepared breakfast, lunch and dinner for us. We only went out to eat on Sundays after church. Occasionally, after piano lessons on Fridays, our family would occasionally go to McDonalds where I could order 2 hamburgers, a small fry and small orange soda for $1.00! (That was several years ago!) However, the majority of the time, we ate food that my mother cooked. We always had a vegetable, rice or potato and a small portion of meat at dinner. A beverage was always consumed after the meal, not with the meal. When we traveled to Norfolk, Va. during the summer, Mommy always packed a meal that we ate in the car. We enjoyed the chicken that she had cooked the night before. We sipped on cool juice while we traveled. Yes, we enjoyed dessert, too!   There wasn't a need to stop at a fast food place along route 95-South, because of Mommy's advanced preparation.

My foundation for nutritional wellness included other things. Mommy never fried our chicken or meats. We were breast-fed as infants. We drank milk that the milkman delivered in a glass bottle. Fruits were our lunch snacks. On occasional Sundays, just before watching "Lassie" on TV, we were treated to a scoop of ice cream with a slice of chocolate layer cake! Our mealtimes around a loving family table included sharing about the activities of our days. Our parents, engaged my sister and me in the art of conversation and family love. We always had grace including thanksgiving to God for having food to eat and praying for those who did not have food to eat. We ate good food in a peaceful, loving home environment.

In all of this, our wonderful mother used to lament that she couldn't cook, just because she didn't prepare "soul food" for us. Soul food was described as the macaroni and cheese made from 4 different types of cheese and other ingredients. Soul food also included fried chicken, fried fish, fried potatoes, barbecued spareribs, chitterlings, sugar-laden desserts etc. Mommy made macaroni and cheese only on some Sundays and on holidays. Her baked macaroni and cheese recipe was simply noodles and cheddar cheese that she carved from a block of cheese. Mommy never fried chicken nor much of anything! She baked our chicken, turkey and we thought it was wonderful. Vegetables and beans (cabbage, collard greens, navy beans, spinach, real corn, cucumbers, and lettuce) that she gave us then are still my favorites today.

When it snowed outside, Mommy left a pan outside to gather the pure, falling snow. We enjoyed the delicious "ice snow" that she made from snow, vanilla and evaporated milk! I thank Mommy today for indeed cooking the best "soul food"....good fuel that nourishes the soul (mind, will and emotions.)!

GEMS for Nutrition Wellness

❖ Eat whole, pure food in a state as close to the way that God created it. For example, if you have the choice between eating organic grapes versus drinking organic grape juice choose to eat organic grapes.

❖ Enjoy food in a non-processed or minimally processed state. For example, eat a baked sweet potato versus eating sweet potato fries. Choose nutrient rich whole grain sprouted flour or brown rice products versus white flour/enriched flour which has been stripped of natural nutrients.

❖ Avoid eating food products that have been made from genetically modified organisms (GMO). For example, corn is one of those vegetables that has been produced from genetically modified seeds. Choose tortilla chips, cereals, products that have the "Non GMO" project verified label on it. Learn more about GMO's from the following online website www.nongmoproject.org

❖ Eat meals in a peaceful environment. Do not eat if there is unrest in your spirit, soul or body.

❖ Chew each bite of food slowly (approximately 25 chews before swallowing the food) to allow the first steps of the digestion process to occur. Food is enjoyed best in the mouth where the taste buds on the tongue allow enjoyment of the food.

❖ Pause and swallow food before placing more food in the mouth. It takes about 20 minutes for the brain to receive the signal that the stomach is satisfied.

❖ When the appetite leaves, because one is ill, listen to that bodily cue! The body is expending tremendous energy fighting the infection and does not need to exert great effort digesting a heavy meal! When the need for more fuel (food) arises, the body will give the hunger signal.

❖ Know your bodily cues for true hunger (stomach growl, it's been 4 or more hours since the last meal, empty feeling in the stomach). If truly hungry, choose wellness attracting whole, pure food.

❖ Avoid overeating. Eat just enough to silence the hunger signal and to give the body time to give the "I'm satisfied" signal.

❖ White sugar (sucrose, high fructose corn syrup) is not a wellness attracting product! White sugar decreases the efficiency of the immune system. White sugar is the "food of choice" for the life of cancer cells. When the desire comes for something sweet, choose to eat a whole fruit (grapes, pineapple, berries, watermelon, apple, raisins, bananas etc.). Organic Agave nectar, in moderation, is a natural substance that is a low-glycemic product (does not cause high spikes in one's blood sugar) that adds natural sweetness to your food. Stevia is another choice.

❖ Stay current with learning about whole food nutrition and healthy living. Some recommended books include: *What Would Jesus Eat* by Dr. Don Colbert, *The Seven Pillars of Health* by Don Colbert, *The Hallelujah Diet* by George Malkmus, *The Wisdom and Healing Power of Whole Foods* by Patrick Quillin, PhD, R.D. Go to www.Forksoverknives.com for healthy recipes ideas and more education about whole food nutrition.

❖ Keep a record of everything that you eat and drink for 24-hours. Prayerfully ask God to confirm a plan of whole-food healthy eating that will benefit your body. Keep a record of everything that you eat and drink for 24 hours. Compare what you've eaten to your God-directed whole-food healthy eating plan.

❖ Variety and color in meal presentation is important. A colorful plate of wellness enhancing food is inviting. Colorful fruits/vegetable/herbs can "spice" up the meals that are served.

❖ Involve young children in the grocery shopping and preparation of meals. Children are likely to eat the vegetables and fruits that they have participated in growing, preparing or buying.

❖ Plant an organic vegetable garden and involve the children/family members in harvesting the vegetables. For those who say, " I don't have space for a garden", consider using the vertical "Tower Garden" sold by Juice Plus (www.juiceplus.com) to grow your fruits and vegetables.

❖ Keep a record of everything that you eat and drink for 24-hours. Prayerfully ask God to confirm a plan of whole-food healthy eating that will benefit your body.

"The doctor of the future will give no medication, but will interest his patients in the care of the human frame, diet and in the cause and prevention of disease."

–Thomas A. Edison

Whole food nutrition is a gem for wellness attraction throughout the lifespan. Pray and ask God to reveal to you His whole food nutrition plan that has been uniquely designed for you.

Detoxification (fasting, proper elimination, avoiding toxins)

Fasting

I remember the first time that I was introduced to fasting as a spiritual discipline. My sister and I as teenagers sang in the choir of our childhood church. The choir director told the choir members, as we approached the choir's anniversary to fast for 24 hours. We did not receive any instruction regarding the "how to" of a fast. However, we trusted that our choir director, who loved the Lord so much, knew what he was talking about. That first 24 hour fast was a water only fast. I don't remember it being a difficult thing to do. I do remember that my spiritual senses were so alive and that I felt so close to God as we celebrated the great things that God had done in our lives!

We live in a world where toxins abound in the environment, household cleaning agents, personal care/beauty products, and in some foods that are consumed. Fasting as a wellness attraction behavior aids the body in cleansing itself of waste. The Bible (The Guide Book for Living) does not say "If you fast" but rather says "When you fast".

17 But when you fast, perfume your head and wash your face,

18 So that your fasting may not be noticed by men but by your Father, Who sees in secret; and your Father, Who sees in secret, will reward you in the open.

Matthew: 6: 17, 18

There are different types of fasts. The absolute fast is going without food or water (not longer than 3 days). This type of fast should only be done under the clear direction of the Holy Spirit. Water only fasts should be done only under the clear direction of the Holy Spirit and with a physician's guidance. The normal fast is going without food but drinking water or liquids for a limited time...1 day, 3 days, 7 days or 40 days. The partial fast is a limited diet in which one abstains from tea, coffee or enjoyable foods (desserts, sugary foods etc.) or skips a meal during a day for a period of time.

How one begins, conducts and ends a fast is critical to the success of the fast. If you are on medications or have a chronic health problem, it is important to consult with your health care provider to determine if fasting is right for you. Do not fast if you are pregnant, nursing or have Type 1 Diabetes.

Pre-Fast GEMS for Wellness Attraction:

- ❖ Pray to determine the purpose of the fast.
- ❖ Pray about the type of fast and how long the fast will be. Beginners should begin with shorter fasts and gradually build up to longer fasts.
- ❖ Schedule your time of personal devotions with God in prayer, praise and worship and reading/meditating on God's Word.
- ❖ Skip the temptation to eat a very large, unhealthy meal just before the fast. Before the start of the fast, begin eating smaller meals. Eat small amounts of easily digestible foods such as fruits and vegetables two days before the fast begins as this helps to prepare the body.

GEMS for Wellness Attraction during the Fast

- ❖ Schedule your day.....When will you have "quiet time" with God in prayer, praise, worship and Bible reading/meditation? Will you have a short prayer walk daily? How can you limit your schedule so that you have times for short power naps? When will you have your juice or eat your partial fast food items?
- ❖ Drink lots of good, pure water during the fast.
- ❖ Avoid chewing gum or mints if you are doing juice fasting. Doing so will cause increased digestive action in your stomach causing you to feel hungrier.
- ❖ Juicing fresh fruits is best, if possible. If you cannot juice fruits or vegetables, purchase 100% fruit or vegetable juices without added sugar or additives.
- ❖ Depending on the length and type of fast, the following symptoms may or may not occur: coated tongue, change in body scent, constipation, headache or irritability. However, after day 3 of the fast (or sometimes sooner), many people report a feeling of heightened spiritual awareness, regularity in having bowel movements, physical healing, increased energy and stamina.

Ending the Fast

- ❖ If you've been fasting for 48 hours or longer on juices only, it is critical that you gently return to eating food. On Day 1, eat small amounts of fruit that have a high water content level as they are easier to digest. On days 2 and 3, add easily-digestible vegetables for lunch and dinner. On day 4, you can add brown rice, warmed soup or a baked potato. By Day 5, organic meat can be added to your meals.

❖ Avoid eating tropical fruits like pineapples and papayas for their strong enzymes could cause stomach upset if eaten in large quantities immediately after the fast.

Recommended Books on Fasting:

The Miracle of Fasting by Paul and Patricia Bragg

Fasting Made Easy by Dr. Don Colbert

The Daniel Fast by Kristen Feola

Fasting: Opening the door to a deeper, more intimate, more powerful relationship with God by Jentezen Franklin

The 40-Day Surrender Fast by Celeste Owens, PhD

The 40-Day Surrender Fast for Kids by A.J. Owens

Fasting for Spiritual Breakthrough by Elmer L. Towns

Proper Elimination

God designed processes in our bodies to eliminate waste. Our respiratory system allows us to breathe in oxygen and eliminate carbon dioxide. Perspiration is released out of the pores of our skin to cool the body. The liver and kidneys are organs of detoxification as well. It is important for us to have daily regular bowel movements for detoxification purposes.

If one consistently eats whole, nutritious food at least 3 times a day, drinks ample water and has an optimally functioning digestive system, one will have 2 to 3 bowel movements a day. What is ingested and digested well should be eliminated. A healthy colon that is not laden with excess waste attracts wellness to the body.

Having a colonic, sometimes called colonic hydration therapy is a process to cleanse and empty the colon. A colon therapist infuses a solution into the rectum which causes the intestines to contract to release stool from the colon. Those who are pregnant, have Crohn's Disease, blood vessel disease, intestinal disease or heart disease should not have a colonic. When I've returned from mission trips abroad, I have had colonic hydrotherapy at a very service excellent business called Enomis Oasis in College Park, Maryland (www.Enomisoasis.com). Others have cleansed their colons using an oral herbal supplement. If you've considered detoxifying your body by having colon hydrotherapy, discuss with your health care provider the pros or cons for you as an individual.

Hydration

Eating well and drinking well are important wellness attraction behaviors. Just as we have choices in what we eat to fuel or bodies, we have choices in what we drink to hydrate our bodies. Water is a great choice for cleansing and hydrating our bodies. The benefits of drinking adequate water include:

- ❖ Water helps to maintain the consistency of vital body fluids. The body is approximately 65% water. Water is in our saliva which aids the first steps of the digestive process. Water is in perspiration which helps in maintaining the temperature of the body. Water is involved in the transport of vital nutrients in the body.
- ❖ Water helps the skin maintain its suppleness.
- ❖ Water aids in the healthy functioning of the cells of the body.
- ❖ Water assists in healthy bowel activity.
- ❖ Water is an effective "aspirin" for those experiencing headaches due to inadequate water intake in relation to fluid output (dehydration).

Remaining hydrated with adequate water is a GEM for wellness attraction.

Rest

And on the seventh day God ended His work which He had done; and He rested on the seventh day from all His work which He had done.

Genesis 2: 2

The sovereign almighty God created the world, all creatures great and small and man/woman in 6 days and rested on the 7th day. There are Biblical accounts of Jesus sleeping. God the Father and God the Son, model for us the necessity of proper REST. If they needed periods of rest, certainly finite man needs to have proper rest.

GEMS for Rest

- ❖ Curtail drinking fluids and engaging in moderate exercise at least 2 hours before bedtime.
- ❖ Create the environment for peaceful sleep. Chamomile tea or warmed milk have been useful to some for inducing sleep.
- ❖ Try to have a consistent time for going to bed and arising whether it's the weekday or weekend.
- ❖ Develop a consistent bedtime routine that alerts your body that it is time to sleep.
- ❖ Meditate on positive scriptures just before going to sleep. (Scriptures: Psalm 23, Psalm 46:10, Psalm 127:2)
- ❖ The aroma of lavender is calming.
- ❖ The immune system functions optimally when one has received enough sleep. Many adults do well with at least 7-8 hours of sleep per night.

Ample periods of rest/rejuvenation is a GEM for Wellness Attraction.

Movement

We were created to move. We have over 650 muscles and 206 bones that assist us in being active. If we couple an exercise like brisk walking with prayer, we've successfully accomplished two gems for wellness attraction...called "prayer walking"!

Benefits of Walking

- ❖ Regular, brisk walking (at least 30 minutes daily) helps in maintaining a healthy weight.
- ❖ Walking as a lifestyle, helps in the prevention and management of health conditions such as heart disease, high blood pressure and diabetes.
- ❖ Brisk walking helps to boost one's mood as endorphins are released into the body.
- ❖ Walking helps with balance and coordination.
- ❖ Regular walking increases blood flow to the brain and has been shown to reduce the incidence of dementia by 40%.
- ❖ Regular walking increases bone strength and density which is particularly important for women. In addition, consistent walking helps in the maintenance of healthy joints which may prevent conditions such as arthritis.
- ❖ Walking strengthens and shapes leg muscles (hamstrings, quadriceps, and calf muscles) lifting gluteal muscles particularly if one walks on an incline.
- ❖ Walking can assist in toning abdominal muscles and whittling the waist, particularly

if one maintains good posture while walking.

❖ If one walks with a walking buddy, this can contribute to relationship building and eliminating feelings of isolation.

❖ Walking outside on a sunny day provides a boost to one's bodily stores of vitamin D—a nutrient that can be difficult to obtain from food, but that can be made from exposure to sunlight.

Developing Your Care Plan for Wellness

2 And the Lord answered me and said, Write the vision and engrave it so plainly upon tablets that everyone who passes May (be able to) read (it easily and quickly as he hastens by.

3For the vision is yet for an appointed time and it hastens to the end (fulfillment); it will not deceive or disappoint. Though it tarry, wait (earnestly) for it, because it will surely come; it will not be behindhand on its appointed day.

Habakkuk 2:2

Every person has been uniquely created in the image of God. Therefore, it is important to be able to understand, the principles of health and wellness that apply specifically to you. We live in an era where there is a plethora of information concerning health and wellness. It is imperative that we pray and ask God for specificity in creating our unique care plan for wellness. One person's immune system functions phenomenally drinking Echinacea tea. Another person may be allergic to it. We have been uniquely created by God. Therefore, take some quiet time and pray and ask God about what should be your unique care plan.

Assessment Phase

❖ How do you practice your faith/religion?

❖ When was the last time that you had a health assessment/medical exam by a physician/nurse practitioner/naturopath/physician assistant?

❖ Do you have any chronic health problems? If so what are they?

❖ Are you currently taking any medications? If so what are they?

❖ What are the biggest challenges that you have experienced or are currently experiencing concerning your spirit, soul or body health?

❖ Are you currently at your desired weight? If not, what things have you tried in order to lose weight?

❖ How would you describe your current nutritional status?

❖ How many hours of sleep do you get most nights of the week?

❖ How many glasses of water do you drink daily?

❖ How much intentional movement do you engage in weekly?

❖ What do you do to manage stress in your life?

❖ What detoxification practices (fasting, colonics) do you practice?

❖ Have you had your blood pressure checked at least once this year?

❖ Are your cholesterol, triglycerides and blood sugar levels normal?

Planning Phase

My Self-Care Plan to Prosper & Be in Health

Wake up time:

Morning Self-care Activities:

Breakfast: (an example of a healthy breakfast you enjoy)

Early afternoon self-care activities:

Healthy Lunch:

Late afternoon self-care activities:

Dinner:

Evening self-care activities:

Bedtime:

New foods/herbs I will try:

New ideas from this book that I will implement:

Health wisdom you received from talking/listening to God:

Implementation Phase

Once you've completed your self-assessment and completed your self-care plan, make a decision to begin implementing at least one wellness attraction behavior as soon as possible. Write down the date of implementation_____

It is said that if you sow a thought it becomes a deed. If you sow a deed it becomes your character. What you sow as your character becomes your destiny! Remember that God placed the gift of prosperity and health into us when we became living souls!

Evaluation Phase

When an action is repeated for at least 21 days it becomes a habit. What one does consistently for 40 days, destroys a stronghold. I welcome hearing your testimony about your path to prosperity and being in health. Send me your testimony at www.Drgaylejones@wellnessattraction.com

Conclusion

You are called nursing colleague to be well in your spirit, soul and body in order to effectively deliver the art of nursing to all in your circle of influence. You are called medical professional to incorporate into your medical practice what Hippocrates said long ago, "Let thy food be your medicine and let thy medicine be food." You are called caregiver of aging parents to put on "your own oxygen mask first" so that you can effectively care for the beloved parent (s) who lovingly cared for you when you were too young to do so. You are called those who want to become pregnant to prepare your bodies to be a healthy "incubator" for forthcoming pregnancies. You are called healthy man or woman to maintain the gift of wellness that God has given you. You are called son or daughter of God to be the light of the world that dispels the darkness that seeks to blanket the Earth and attempt to steal the gift of health given to us by God. You are called college freshman to be a doer of all the wisdom that you received while at home regarding living well. The "Freshman Fifteen" (weight gain) does not have to be your destiny! You are called, to reverse pre-diabetes to "no diabetes" as you choose a radically different lifestyle of wellness. You are called to hear that the flu is around but does not have to be in you! You are called pastor, minister, church leader, Christian man or woman to walk the talk of living the abundant life (John 10:10) that Jesus purchased for us through His death.

It is my prayer that you heard the voice of Jesus speaking clearly to you as in John 10:10..."I have come that they may have life and that more abundantly." You can prosper and be in health! Be a G.E.M. (God's Excellent Model) and shine brilliantly with wellness in your spirit, soul and body!

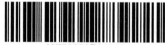

49779358R00030

Made in the USA
Charleston, SC
04 December 2015